PRACTICAL ENGLISH FOR DIETITIANS
REVISED EDITION

Shigeko Ogawa   Atsuko Yamamoto   Laura Nihan

GAKKEN SHOIN

● はじめに ●

　このテキストは，2000年に発行されたPRACTICAL ENGLISH FOR DIETITIANSの改訂新版です．第2版を受けついで，栄養士の活動にかかわるさまざまな英語表現を紹介していますが，このたびまったく新しい資料をもとに，内容を再編成いたしました．

　Chapter 1 は，英語でレシピを読み，自分でも実際に書いて発表できるように，という構成です．調理用語，食材名，数量表現などを自由に組み合わせてみましょう．現代の健康志向に合わせ，適切な食材を選ぶこともねらいにしています．

　Chapter 2 のテーマは，食品衛生です．食中毒予防のための注意事項などを，わかりやすくクイズ形式で紹介しましたので，挑戦してみてください．さらに食材の取り扱いに関する専門用語や，おもな食中毒分類表なども掲載しました．温度表示や医学用語にもふれています．

　Chapter 3 では，老化予防，10代の食生活など，日常でも話題になるテーマについて，栄養素名や生活習慣病にかかわる英文を読む構成になっています．やや長い文もありますが，ページわきに簡単な用語解説をつけました．関心のあるパラグラフを拾って読んだり，exercise で確認しながら読むなど，根気よく取り組んでみましょう．

　Chapter 4 は，初版以来このテキスト編集にご指導いただいてきたローラ・ナイアンさんが，メッセージをおくってくださいました．栄養士の先輩としてだけでなく，みなさんのこれからの人生への心のこもった応援歌です．さらにステップアップをめざす際のツールについて，くわしく紹介されています．なお，ナイアンさんは日本での教員経験もお持ちです．とくに栄養士をめざす学生への関心や熱意は，この Chapter を通じてもご理解いただける

ことと思います．今回も全編にわたり監修をお願いいたしました．

　Appendix には，今後の栄養士業務に役立つと思われる臓器のイラスト，栄養素とその供給源，体内での働きなどについての図表をのせました．各 Chapter を学習するときの参考にしてください．

　みなさんは今後，栄養士として，多くの国の人々と，食物や栄養について話す機会も増えることでしょう．このテキストの内容がコミュニケーションの道具として役立てば幸いです．

　最後に，ナイアンさん来日にあたり，American Overseas Dietetic Association 日本代表である管理栄養士 芹澤ともみさんにも，連絡役として，また助手として，ご協力いただきました．お礼申し上げます．

　さらに，このテキストの初版から，長年にわたり見守ってくださっている学建書院大崎真弓編集部長，そして実に根気よく実務万端をリードし，改訂新版の誕生に立ち会ってくださった編集担当馬島めぐみさんに，心から感謝の意を表します．

2010 年 4 月

小川成子

山本厚子

Laura Nihan

CONTENTS

Chapter 1
LET'S MAKE SALADS! 1

Chapter 2
FOOD SAFETY 13

Chapter 3
OUR BODY AND NUTRITION 25

Chapter 4
DIETITIAN'S MESSAGE 57

APPENDIX 65

Chapter 1

LET'S MAKE SALADS !

Match the names.

carrots

cucumbers

tomatoes

pumpkins

eggplants

green peppers

cabbage

MIXED SALAS !

MIXED SALAD

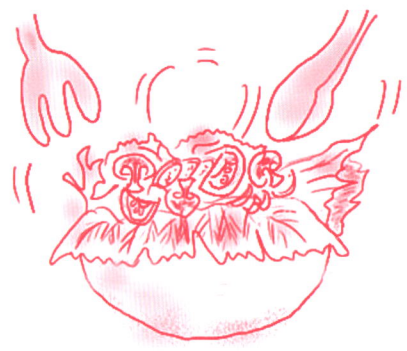

Ingredients

2 cucumbers, sliced
3 medium tomatoes, diced
1 celery stalk, sliced
1/2 onion, thinly sliced
1 green pepper, cut into strips
lettuce leaves
1 egg, boiled and cut into 4 wedges

(*Serves 4*)

French dressing (recipe follows)

Directions

1 Put the cucumber, tomato, celery, green pepper and onion into the bowl, and toss.
2 Place lettuce leaves on a platter, and arrange the tossed vegetables on them.
3 Garnish with egg wedges on top : cover and chill.

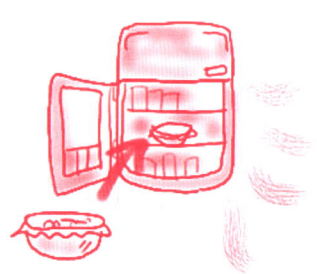

French Dressing : *Makes 1 1/2 cups*

1/2 tsp salt	1/2 tsp sugar
1/4 tsp pepper	2 Tbsp white vinegar
1/2 tsp dry mustard	1 cup salad oil

Put all the dry ingredients into a bottle. Pour the vinegar and stir. Add the oil and shake until well blended.

Terms for Preparation (1)

C : cup…1 cup, 1 1/2 cups, 4 cups...
Tbsp : tablespoon…1/2 Tbsp, 1 1/4 tablespoons...
tsp : teaspoon…1/3 teaspoon, 6 teaspoons...

Terms for Preparation (2)

whole ↔ cut into ┬ strips
                 ├ half, halves
                 └ wedges

chop, slice, shred, dice

finely—roughly, thinly

POTATO SALAD

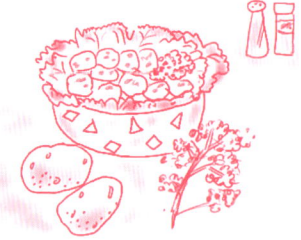

450 g potatoes, cooked and diced
100 g carrots, cooked and diced
1/2 C, canned green peas, drained
1/2 C, canned kernel corn, drained
1/2 medium onion, finely chopped
2/3 C mayonnaise
1 Tbsp, chopped parsley
salt and pepper to taste
salad green

1. Combine the cooked potatoes, boiled carrots and chopped onion with mayonnaise.
2. Add peas and corn. Season with salt and pepper to taste.
3. Place salad greens around the edge of a salad bowl, and spoon the mixture into the center.
4. Garnish with parsley. Chill until served.

(Serves 4)

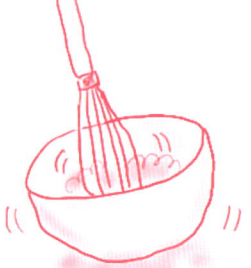

——— *Terms for Preparation* (3) ———

fresh ↔ cooked
fresh ↔ dried, canned, frozen, preserved, etc.

STRAWBERRY SURPRISE

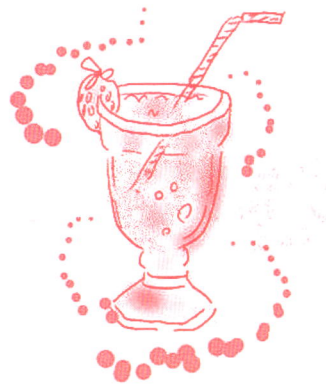

Ingredients
3/4 C low-fat milk
1/2 package strawberries
1/2 C strawberry yogurt
pinch cinnamon

(Makes 1 cup)

Utensils
Measuring cups
Blender or food processor
Glasses to serve

This drink is so thick, it could be eaten as a dessert or snack. Try bananas, peaches, or any of your favorite fruits for different flavors.

Directions
1. Remove stems from the strawberries.
2. Pour milk into blender.
3. Put the strawberries into the blender. Add the strawberry yogurt.
4. Put the lid on the blender. Blend well until thick and frothy.
5. Pour into glasses and chill until served. Sprinkle cinnamon.

GOT LEFTOVERS ?

CHICKEN SOUP

1 Heat 1 Tbsp oil in a medium saucepan over medium-high heat. Add 1 small diced onion and 1 sliced celery stalk ; cook for 5 minutes, or until browned.

2 Pour in 1 can (48 oz) chicken broth and heat to boil.

3 Add 1 1/2 cups shredded cooked chicken, and 1 cup each shredded carrot and cooked egg noodles ; heat thoroughly. Season to taste with salt and pepper, and serve hot !

——— **Terms for Cooking** ———

cook : cook, boil, steam, simmer
　　　　fry, stir-fry, deep-fry
bake : bake, grill, roast
microwave

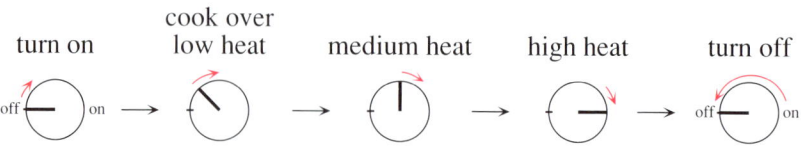

TRY SOME BAKING !

When you make cakes, cookies, and breads **with an oven**, it is **not cooking** : it is **baking**.

CUTOUT HOLIDAY COOKIES (*Makes 12-14 cookies*)

125 g butter	2 tsp imitation vanilla essence
1/3 cup sugar	2 cups plain flour
1 egg yolk	1 Tbsp raisins, finely chopped

1 Turn oven to 160°C.

2 Beat butter, sugar, egg yolk and vanilla in a small bowl until light and creamy.

3 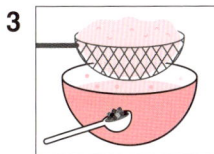 Sift flour into bowl. Add raisins. Mix to a soft dough. **4** 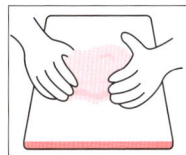 Knead gently on a lightly-floured board.

5 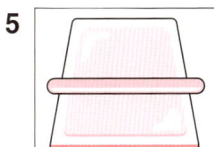 Roll out thinly. **6** 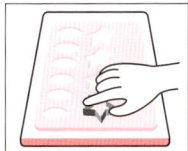 Cut dough into shapes.

7 Bake on top shelf for 20 minutes.

MUFFINS

1 Mix 1/2 cup mashed sweet potato with 1/3 cup buttermilk. Combine 2 1/4 cups all-purpose baking mix with potato mixture and another 1/3 cup buttermilk.

2 Mix to form dough. Knead 12 times on a surface coated with the baking mix. Roll out to 1/2 in. ; cut into rounds. Bake on an ungreased baking pan for 10 minutes in a 450°F oven.

FETTUCCINE AND SPINACH BAKE

Prep time : 35 minutes
Start to finish : 1 hour
Servings : 6

> ■ Nutrition information per serving ■
> Calories 490 (calories from Fat 220),
> Total Fat 25 g (Saturated Fat 14 g),
> Cholesterol 115 mg ; Sodium 860 mg ;
> Total Carbohydrate 51g (Dietary Fiber 5 g ;
> Sugars 8 g) ; Protein 16 g

1 package (12 oz) uncooked fettuccine
2 tablespoons butter
1 medium-sized onion, chopped (1/2 cup)
2 cloves garlic, finely chopped
1/2 teaspoon salt
2 cans (14.5 oz) stewed tomatoes, undrained
1 bag (1lb) frozen cut-leaf spinach, thawed and squeezed to drain
1 cup shredded Swiss cheese (4 oz)

1 Preheat oven to 400 ℉.
2 Cook and drain fettuccine as directed on package.
3 Melt butter in 10-inch skillet.
  Put onion and cook 3 to 4 minutes, stir frequently until tender. Add garlic, salt, and both cans of tomatoes. Add basil and oregano, and cook for 5 min. Stir occasionally until tomatoes are hot.
4 In an ungreased 13×9-inch glass baking dish, spread half of the fettuccine. Layer with all of the spinach and half of the tomato mixture. Repeat with the remaining fettuccine and tomato mixture.
5 Pour cream over top ; sprinkle evenly with cheese.
6 Bake uncovered for 20 to 25 minutes until hot, and cheese is melted.

Terms for Preparation (4)

F (Fahrenheit) $=9/5\ C+32$
C (Centigrade or Celsius) $=5/9\ (F-32)$
　　　　medium heat ： 180 °C＝360 °F
　　　　very high heat： 240 °C＝480 °F

Terms for Preparation (5)

drained	↔	undrained
frozen	↔	thawed
frequently	↔	occasionally
greased	↔	ungreased
covered	↔	uncovered

Terms for Preparation (6)

1 lb (pound) ＝450 g
1 oz (ounce) ＝1/16 lb＝28 g
1 inch＝2.5 cm

Pasta Varieties

long pasta： capellini, vermicelli, fettuccine, spaghettini, linguine
short pasta： macaroni, penne
others： ravioli, lasagna, gnocchi, cannelloni, etc.,

STIR CRAZY

With our mix-and-match plan,
your tasty stir-fry possibilities are endless.

Getting started

Make a **sauce**, below, then select **protein**, **vegetables**, **sides** and *finishing touches* to complete the meal.

Sauces

A PEANUT	B GINGER-SOY
Whisk 1 cup water, 1/3 cup creamy peanut butter, 2 Tbsp reduced-sodium soy sauce*, 2 tsp minced garlic and 1/4 tsp crushed red pepper in small bowl until blended.	Stir 1/2 cup orange juice, 1/4 cup reduced-sodium soy sauce, 2 Tbsp water, 1 Tbsp grated ginger, 1 tsp cornstarch and 1 tsp sesame oil in small bowl until cornstarch is dissolved**.

*reduced-sodium soy sauce：減塩しょう油（sodium：Na）

**dissolve：(液体中に) 溶かす，溶ける　　　cf. melt：(熱で) 溶かす，溶ける

How to cook

1. Put 2 Tbsp cornstarch and 1 lb **protein** into a large ziptop bag, seal bag and shake to coat.
2. Heat 1 Tbsp oil in large nonstick skillet. Add **protein**; stir-fry over medium-high heat for 3 to 5 minutes until thoroughly cooked. Remove to a serving plate.
3. Add 2 tsp oil to skillet; heat. Add 4 cups of any one of combinations of **vegetables**; stir-fry for 3 to 5 minutes until crisp-tender.
4. Add sauce to skillet; bring to simmer. Add **protein**; simmer for 1 to 2 minutes until sauce thickens and coats the mixture.
5. Serve with choice of **side**, and top with *finishing touches*.

LET'S MAKE SALADS !

Protein (1 LB)

- peeled and drained shrimps
- boneless, skinless chicken breasts, cut into 1.5 cm thick cubes
- sliced beef or pork, cut into 5 cm
- firm tofu (*momen*), cut into 2.5 cm cubes

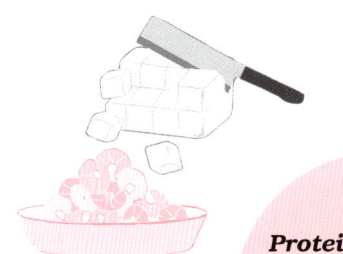

Vegetables (4 CUPS)

- small broccoli florets
- 1 cm thick red onion wedges
- small cauliflower florets
- thinly sliced carrots
- sliced *shiitake* mushrooms
- asparagus, cut into 3 cm
- cooked *edamame*
- snow peas
- red or yellow peppers, cut into 1.5 cm-long strips

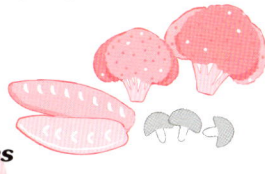

Finishing Touches

- cashews, peanuts or almonds
- finely chopped *konegi*
- roasted sesame seeds
- chopped *mitsuba*
- cayenne pepper
- vinegar

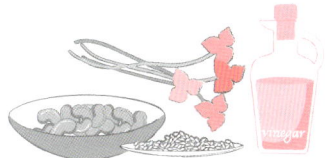

Sides (Carbohydrates)

- cooked brown rice
- cooked wholegrain rice
- buckwheat noodles, boiled
- *harusame* noodles, boiled
- Chinese noodles for stir-fry

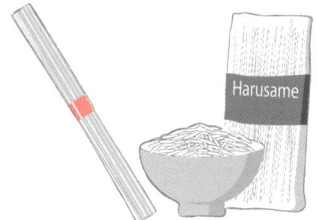

List of the Food

Meat
- lamb — mutton
- veal — beef
- pork

Poultry
- chicken
- turkey
- goose
- duck

Seafood
- fish   freshwater fish ; salmon, trout, eel
                seawater fish ; sardine, cod, sole, tuna
- shellfish   shrimp — prawn — lobster
                   (large shrimp)
              crab
              clam, oyster, scallop abalone
- octopus, squid
- seaweed

—— Kitchen Utensils ——

pan   kettle   skillet   microwave oven

blender   grater   drainer   food processor

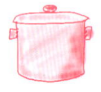 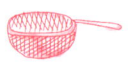 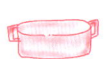

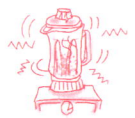 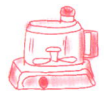

Chapter 2

FOOD SAFETY

Four Simple Steps to Food Safety

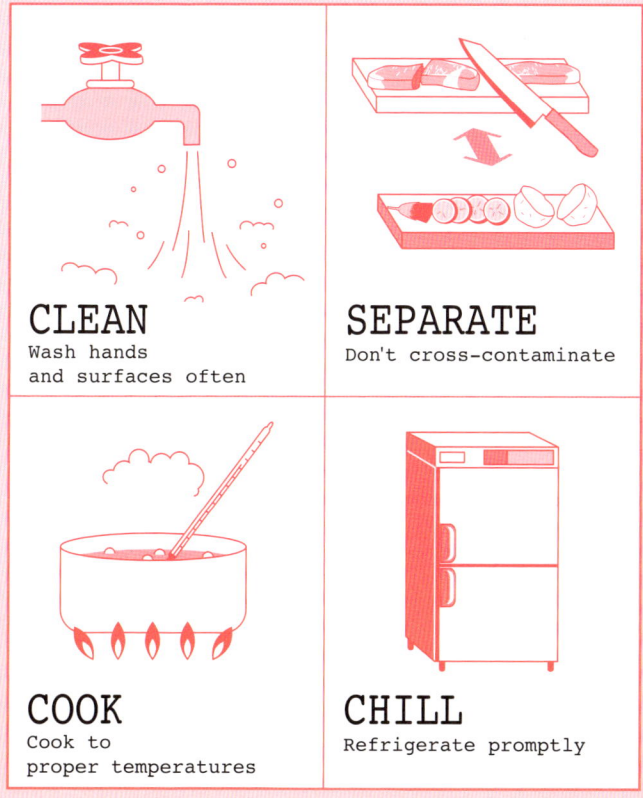

Keep Food Safe From Bacteria

1 FOUR KEYS TO SAFER FOOD

Fill in the blanks. Change if necessary.

1. KEEP CLEAN

- Wash your hands before (①   ) food and often during food preparation.
- Wash your hands after (②   ) to the toilet.
- Wash and sanitize₁₎ all surfaces and equipment (③   ) for food preparation.
- (④   ) kitchen areas and food from insects, pests₂₎ and other animals.

《 use   handle   go   protect 》

2. SEPARATE RAW AND COOKED

- Separate raw₃₎ meat, (⑤   ) and seafood from other foods.
- Use separate equipment and (⑥   ) such as knives and cutting boards for handling raw foods.
- Store food in (⑦   ) to avoid contact between raw and prepared foods.

《 utensils₄₎   poultry₅₎   containers 》

FOOD SAFETY

1. Why ?

While most microorganisms[6] do not cause disease, dangerous microorganisms are widely found in soil, water, animals, and people. These microorganisms are carried on hands, wiping cloths and utensils, especially cutting boards, and the slightest contact can transfer them to food and cause foodborne diseases[7].

2. Why ?

Raw food, especially meat, poultry and seafood and their juices, can contain dangerous microorganisms which may be transferred onto other foods during food preparation and storage.

■ note ■

1) sanitize : to clean something thoroughly, removing dirt and bacteria
2) pest (s) : a small animal or insect that harms people or destroys things
3) raw : not cooked
4) utensil : a tool or object with a particular use, especially in cooking
5) poultry : birds such as chickens and ducks kept on farms for supplying eggs and meat
6) microorganism : a living thing that is so small that it cannot be seen without a microscope
7) foodborne disease : an illness caused by eating food that contains harmful bacteria, resulting in symptoms such as diarrhea or vomiting

3. COOK THOROUGHLY

- (⑧   ) food thoroughly, especially meat, poultry, eggs and seafood.
- Bring foods like soups and stews to boiling to make sure that they have (⑨   ) 70 °C. For meat and poultry, make sure that juices (⑩   ) clear, not pink. Ideally, use a thermometer₁).
- (⑪   ) cooked food thoroughly.

《 be   reach   cook   reheat 》

4. KEEP FOOD AT SAFE TEMPERATURES

- Do not (⑫   ) cooked food at room temperature for more than 2 hours.
- Refrigerate promptly all cooked and (⑬   ) food (preferably below 5 °C)
- Keep cooked food piping hot (more than 60 °C) before (⑭   ).
- Do not (⑮   ) food too long even in the refrigerator.
- Do not (⑯   ) frozen food at room temperature.

《 store   serve   thaw₂)   perish₃)   leave 》

16

FOOD SAFETY

3. Why ?

Proper cooking can kill almost all dangerous microorganisms. Studies have shown that cooking food to a temperature of 70 °C can help ensure it is safe for consumption[4]. Foods that require special attention include minced meats, rolled roasts, large joints of meat and whole poultry.

4. Why ?

Microorganisms can multiply[5] very quickly if food is stored at room temperature. By holding at temperatures below 5 °C or above 60 °C, the growth of microorganisms is slowed down or stopped. Some dangerous microorganisms still grow below 5 °C.

■ n o t e ■

1) thermometer : equipment that measures the temperature of air, food or your body
2) thaw : to defrost, or to let frozen food unfreeze until it is ready to cook
3) perish (perishable) : the food that is likely to decay if it is not kept in the correct conditions
4) consumption : the act of eating or drinking, or the amount of food or drink one consumes
5) multiply : to increase greatly

《Answers》

① handling ② going ③ used ④ Protect ⑤ poultry ⑥ utensils ⑦ containers ⑧ Cook ⑨ reached ⑩ are ⑪ Reheat ⑫ leave ⑬ perishable ⑭ serving ⑮ store ⑯ thaw

2　FATTOM MNEMONIC

Describes conditions needed for bacteria to grow.
Bacteria grow best when they have······

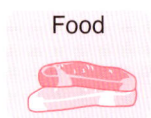
Food

Foods high in protein and carbohydrate

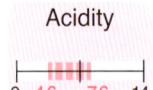
Acidity

Acidity with a pH between 4.6 to 7.6

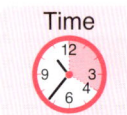
Time

Temperature 41°F to 135°F
Time-no more than four hours in the temperature danger zone*(5°C and 57°C)

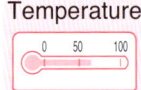
Temperature

*Note：It is also allowable to bring food from 135°F to 70°F within two(2)hours and from 70°F to 41°F within an additional four(4)hours.

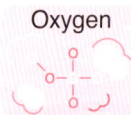
Oxygen

Oxygen for some bacteria and no oxygen for others (aerobic or anaerobic)

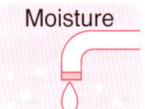
Moisture

Moisture levels of ≧0.85 Aw
Aw is defined as water activity···the amount of available water in food. Bacteria will grow at an Aw level as low as 0.85, however, most bacteria grow at a level of 0.97～0.99.
Bacteria double in number every 20 minutes. The growth slows at 32°F(0°C), but the bacteria are not killed. Darkness causes bacteria to multiply.

3   FOOD HOLDING

- Hold cold foods below 41°F (5 °C).
- Hold hot foods above 135°F (57 °C).
- Never mix new food with old food.
- Regularly stir foods during holding.
- Measure food temperature every 2 hours.
- Cover holding pans and provide long handled serving utensils.
- Use good food handling procedures during service.

63°C = 145°F
68°C = 155°F
74°C = 165°F

◆ **EXERCISES** ◆

(1) Explain the following.
   1) danger zone
   2) two-hour rules
(2) Why do we use long-handled serving utensils ?
(3) Which is more preferable condition for food handling ?
   1) Aw level : 0.73 or 0.92
   2) in darkness or in light places

◆ **ANSWERS** ◆

(1)
   1) between 5 °C and 57 °C
   2) Perishable foods should not be left at room temperature longer than two hours.
(2) Harmful bacteria can be transferred from hands to foods. The longer the distance between hands and foods, the better.
(3)
   1) Aw level : 0.73 (bacteria will grow at an Aw level as low as 0.85)
   2) Darkness causes bacteria to multiply.

4 MAJOR FOODBORNE ILLNESSES CAUSED BY BACTERIA

Most Important Prevention Measure			Controlling time and temperature
Illness			***Bacillus cereus*** gastroenteritis
Bacteria Characteristics	Commonly Linked Food	Poultry	
		Eggs	
		Meat	○
		Fish	
		Shellfish	
		Ready-to-eat food	
		Produce	○
		Rice/grains	○
		Milk/dairy products	○
		Contaminated water	
	Most Common Symptoms	Diarrhea[1]	○
		Abdominal pain/cramps[2]	
		Nausea[3]	○
		Vomiting[4]	○
		Fever	
		Headache	
	Prevention Measures	Handwashing	
		Cooking	○
		Holding	○
		Cooling	○
		Reheating	
		Approved suppliers	
		Excluding foodhandlers	
		Preventing cross-contamination[5]	

FOOD SAFETY

Controlling time and temperature			
Listeriosis	Hemorrhagic colitis	***Clostridium perfringens*** gastroenteritis	Botulism
		○	
○	○	○	
○			
	○		○
○			
	○	○	
	○	○	
			○
			○
○	○		
		○	○
		○	○
		○	○
	○		
	○		
○	○		

21

FOOD SAFETY

Most Important Prevention Measure			Preventing cross-contamination
Illness			Salmonellosis
Bacteria Characteristics	Commonly Linked Food	Poultry	○
		Eggs	○
		Meat	
		Fish	
		Shellfish	
		Ready-to-eat food	
		Produce	○
		Rice/grains	
		Milk/dairy products	○
		Contaminated water	
	Most Common Symptoms	Diarrhea[1]	○
		Abdominal pain/cramps[2]	○
		Nausea[3]	
		Vomiting[4]	○
		Fever	○
		Headache	
	Prevention Measures	Handwashing	
		Cooking	○
		Holding	
		Cooling	
		Reheating	
		Approved suppliers	
		Excluding foodhandlers	○
		Preventing cross-contamination[5]	○

FOOD SAFETY

Practicing personal hygiene[6]		Purchasing from approved, reputable suppliers
Shigellosis	Staphylococcal gastroenteritis	*Vibrio vulnificus primary* septicemia/gastroenteritis
		○
○	○	
○		
○		○
○		○
○	○	○
	○	○
	○	○
○		○
○	○	
		○
	○	
	○	
	○	
		○
○		

■ note ■

1) diarrhea [dàiərí:ə]：下痢. (cf) loose bowels [báuəl]
2) abdominal [æbdámən(ə)l] pain/cramps：激しい腹痛.
3) nausea [nɔ́:ziə,-ʃə] 吐き気.
4) vomiting [vámətiŋ]：嘔吐.
5) cross-contamination：相互汚染.
6) hygiene [háidʒi:n]：衛生，清潔.

Chapter 3

OUR BODY AND NUTRITION

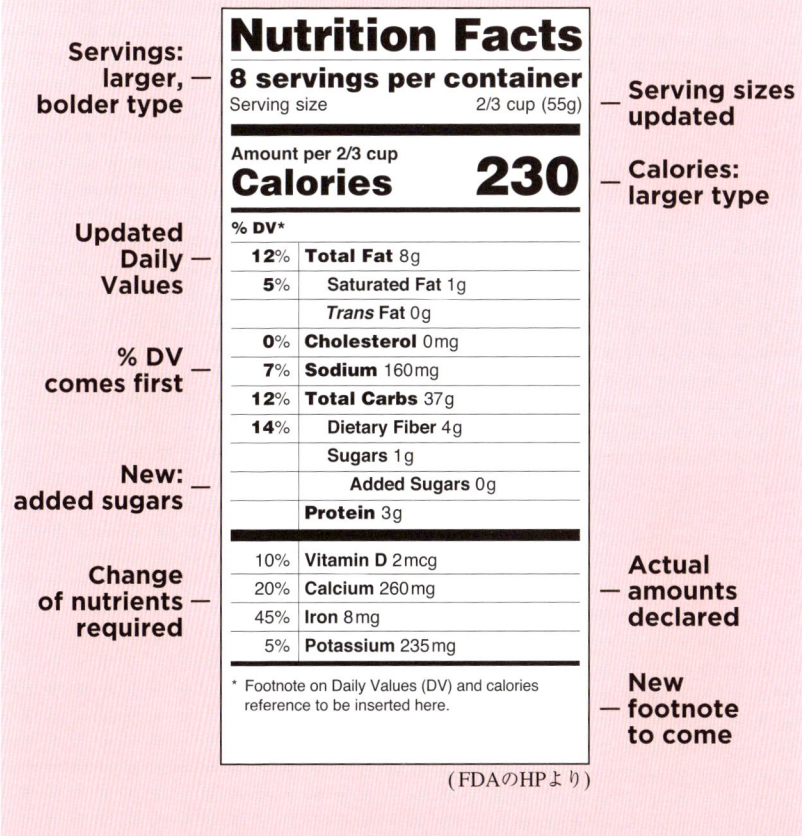

(FDAのHPより)

1 WHAT TEENS TYPICALLY EAT IN A DAY
WHAT THEY SHOULD BE EATING INSTEAD

TOO MANY CALORIES
Taking in over 3,000 calories a day is too much for most teens.

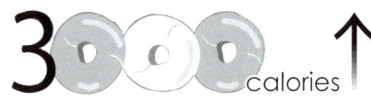

FEWER CALORIES
Except for those who exercise vigorously, 2,600~2,700 is the target range.

NOT ENOUGH CALCIUM
As intake of soft drinks goes up, calcium consumption[1] goes down. This is worrisome since half of the bone mass[2] as adults is formed during the teen years.

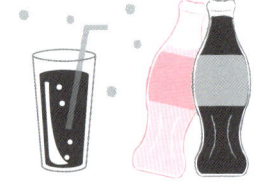

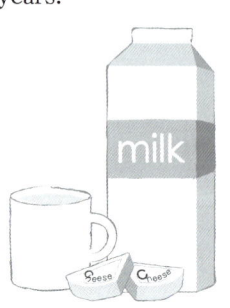

MORE CALCIUM
Some teens are getting a healthy dose of calcium mainly from low-fat cheese and milk. By eliminating[3] soft drinks from the diet, the amount of phosphorus[4], which can cause calcium loss, is dramatically reduced[5].

Ans. 1) milk, cheese, yogurt, for example. 2) half/mass/teen

1) Give three names of food which are rich in calcium.
   ( ), ( ), ( )
2) Why is calcium so important for teens' everyday meals?
   Because ( ) of the bone ( ) as adults is formed during the ( ) years.

26

OUR BODY AND NUTRITION

NOT ENOUGH FIBER
Teens need about 30g of fiber for sustained energy, normal digestion and reduced risk of cancer. The more highly processed foods kids eat, the less fiber they take in from whole grains, fruits and vegetables.

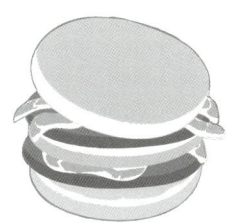

TOO FEW FRUITS AND VEGGIES
Only a few items (fries, chips) even come close to counting as a fruit or vegetable, and they are high in sugar or fat. And these foods are not what USDA had in mind with the "five a day" recommendation.

MORE FIBER, FRUITS AND VEGETABLES
Replacing the bagel with a whole-wheat[6] bun and multigrain cereal, and adding more fresh fruits and vegetables throughout the menu, bring the day's intake into a healthy range (46 g).

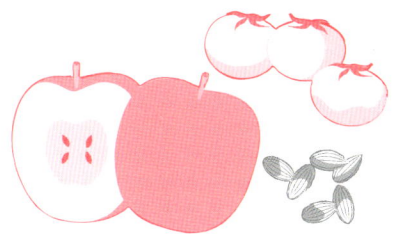

1) In order to take enough fiber, recommend five kinds of vegetables and fruits for your family.
 (　　), (　　), (　　), (　　), (　　)
2) Let's try to take more (　　) bread and (　　) cereal, instead of white bread, and add more fresh (　　) and foods low in (　　), to make your everyday diet more healthful.

Ans. 1) Rf. Chapter 1　2) whole-wheat/multigrain/fruits and vegetables/sugar or fat

27

TOO MUCH FAT
Only 30% (about 90g) of children's total calories should come from fat and just 10% from saturated fats[7] such as those found in meat and cheese products.

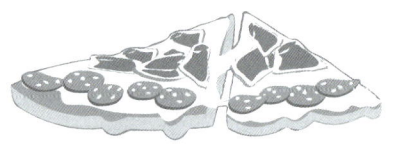

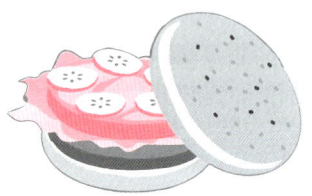

BETTER FAT
If some vegetable toppings are added, a turkey burger and rice pudding could cut down the fat almost 50%. Saturated fat is slashed even more with this method.

A MOUND OF SUGAR
About 43 teaspoons can be found in soft drinks, ice cream and other sweets. To prevent obesity[8], no more than 10% of teen's daily calories (only 50 to 70g) should come from added sugar.

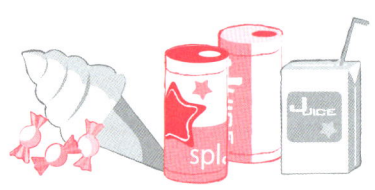

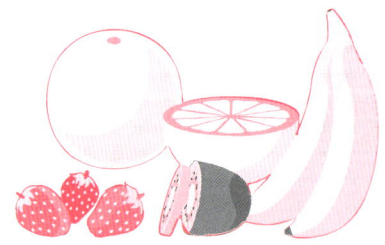

LESS SUGAR
Doing away with sweet beverages drops the total sugar in this daily menu down to 112g. That's still high, but most of the sugar obtained in this meal is natural, found in fruit and other foods.

1) About (　) of children's total calories should come from (　), and only 10% from (　) fats such as those found in meat and cheese.
2) If you stop drinking (　), the total sugar in such fast food meals is reduced greatly.

Ans. 1) 1/3(or 30%)/fat/saturated 2) sweet beverages

OUR BODY AND NUTRITION

AN INFUSION OF SALT
About three-quarters of the sodium in teens' diets shows up in prepared or processed foods (like French fries). Only about 11% is added during cooking or via the saltshaker at the table.

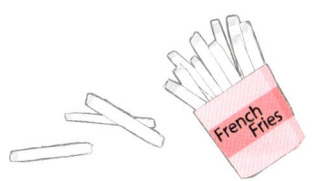

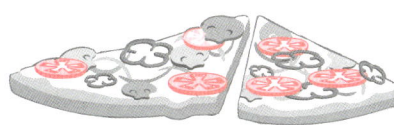

LESS SODIUM
Reduced by about a third, a fast food menu still has more sodium than the recommended amount. Eating more meals at home prepared with fresh[9] ingredients is a great way to keep sodium levels under control.

Ans.　1) three　2) sodium/meals

1) A fast food menu has more than (　　) times of the recommended amount for sodium.
2) "Prepared or processed foods" include various canned or frozen ingredients, while more fresh ingredients are used at home. You can control (　　) level much easier by eating more (　　) prepared at home.

■ note ■

1) consumption：消費量（↔intake）．
2) bone mass：骨量，骨中のミネラル分の量．
3) eliminate：除去する，排出する．
4) phosphorus：リン．
5) reduce：減らす，減少させる．
6) whole-wheat：(小麦，とうもろこしなどの) 全粒．
7) saturated fat：飽和脂肪酸 (↔unsaturated fat)
8) obesity：肥満症．
9) fresh：生の，(缶詰や冷凍，乾燥，塩漬などの) 加工をされていない．

29

2　ACS GUIDELINES for CANCER PREVENTION

■　n o t e　■

1) obese ［oubíːs］：肥満の
 (cf. obesity ; (病的) 肥満, overweight ; 過体重).

2) menopause：更年期.

3) colon ［kóulən］：結腸, 大腸.

4) kidney：腎臓.

　This document is the condensed and modified article describing the American Cancer Society Nutrition and Physical Guidelines. The full article, written for health care professionals, is published in 2006, and is available for free online at：http：// caonline.amcancersoc.org/content/vol56/issues5/.

Maintain a Healthy Weight throughout Life

　In order to maintain a healthy weight throughout life, balance calorie intake with physical activity, avoid excessive weight gain, and achieve and maintain a healthy weight if currently overweight or obese[1].

　Being overweight or obese is clearly linked with an increased risk of developing several types of cancer, such as breast（among women who have gone through menopause[2]）, colon[3], esophagus, or kidney[4]. Obesity is also likely to raise the risk of other cancers, as gallbladder, ovary, pancreas, and others. While research in this area is still going on, people who are overweight or obese are encouraged to lose weight.

A healthy weight depends on a person's height, so recommendations for a healthy weight are often expressed by body mass index (BMI). BMI is a measure of body fat based on height and weight. (*See page 32.*)

Adopt a Physically Active Lifestyle

Usual activities are those that are done as part of one's daily routine, at work, at home, or as part of daily living. Usual activities are typically brief and of low intensity. Intentional activities are done in addition to these usual activities. Moderate activities require effort equal to a brisk walk. Vigorous activities generally use large muscle groups and cause faster heart rate, deeper and faster breathing, and sweating. The benefits of a physically active lifestyle go far beyond lowering cancer risk. They include lower risk of heart disease, high blood pressure, diabetes[1], and osteoporosis[2] (bone thinning).

Eat a Healthy Diet, with an Emphasis on Plant Sources.

Choose foods and beverages in amounts that help achieve and maintain a healthy weight. Eat

---

■ note ■

1) diabetes [daiəbíːtiz]：糖尿病.

2) osteoporosis [ɑstioupəróusəs]：(*u*) a disease in which the bones become very weak and break easily.

Are You at a Healthy Weight?

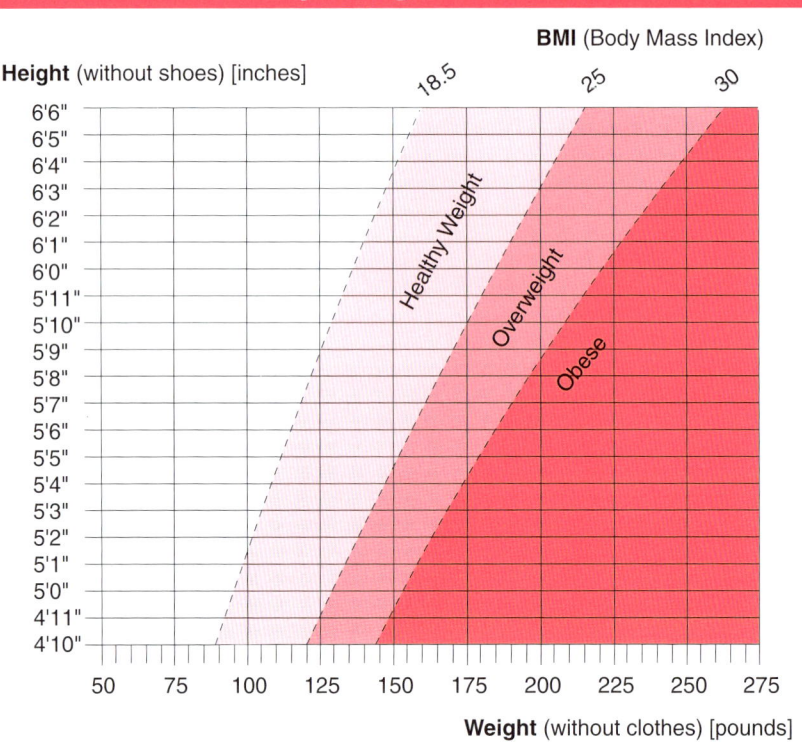

Height (without shoes) [inches]

BMI (Body Mass Index)

Weight (without clothes) [pounds]

The BMI ranges shown above are for adults. They are not exact ranges of healthy and unhealthy weights. However, they show that health risk increase at higher levels of overweight and obesity. Even within the healthy BMI range, weight gains can carry health risks for adults.

Directions : Find your weight on the bottom of the graph. Go straight up from that point until you come to the line that matches your height. Then look to find your weight group.

- **Healthy Weight** : BMI from 18.5 up to 25 refers to healthy weight.
- **Overweight** : BMI from 25 up to 30 refers to overweight.
- **Obese** : BMI 30 or higher refers to obesity. Obese persons are also overweight.

(Source : Report of the Dietary Guidelines Advisory Committee on the Dietary Guidelines for Americans, 2000.)

OUR BODY AND NUTRITION

smaller portions of high-calorie foods. Be aware that "low-fat" or "non-fat" does not mean "low-calorie". Switch to vegetables, fruits and other low-calorie foods and beverages to replace calorie-dense foods and beverages. Eat 5 or more varieties of vegetables and fruits each day. Include vegetables and fruits at every meal and for snacks. Choose 100% juice if you drink vegetable or fruit juices.

Choose whole grains[1] over processed (refined[2]) grains and sugars. Limit intake of refined carbohydrates[3] (starches), such as pastries, sweetened cereals, and other high-sugar foods. Limit intake of processed meats and red meats. Choose fish, poultry[4], or beans instead of beef, pork, and lamb. When you eat meat, choose lean[5] cuts and eat smaller portions.

Eating processed meats, preserved with nitrites[6], smoke or salt, increases exposure[7] to potential cancer-causing agents and should be reduced as much as possible. Prepare meat by baking, broiling, or poaching, rather than by frying, or charbroiling.

If you drink alcoholic beverages, limit your intake. People who drink alcohol should limit

■ note ■

1) whole grains：未精製の穀類．

2) refined：精製された．

3) carbohydrate [kɑː(r)bouháidreit]：炭水化物．

4) poultry [póultri]：birds such as chickens and ducks kept on farms．

5) lean [líːn]：脂肪の少ない，赤身の．

6) nitrite [náitrait]：亜硝酸塩．

7) exposure：the state of being put into a harmful or bad situation without having any protection. 曝露（病原菌などにさらされること）．

note

1) folate : 葉酸.
 ref. p. 47~54

their intake to no more than 2 drinks per day for men and 1 drink a day for women. The recommended limit is lower for women because of their smaller body size and slower breakdown of alcohol. The combination of alcohol and tobacco increases the risk of some cancers far more than the effect of either drinking or smoking alone. Regular intake of even a few drinks per week is linked to a higher risk of breast cancer in women, especially in women who do not get enough folate[1]. Alcohol is a known cause of colon cancer. Some studies show a lower risk of colon cancer among those who are moderately active ; obesity raises the risk of colon cancer in both men and women, but the link seems to be stronger in men. Diets high in processed meats and/or red meats have been linked with a higher risk of colon cancer.

Common Questions about Diet and Cancer

Since people are interested in the relationship between specific foods, nutrients, or lifestyle and specific cancers, research on health behaviors and cancer risk is often reported on the news.

No one study, however, provides the last word on any subject, and single news reports may put too much emphasis on what appear to be contradictory or conflicting results[1]. The following questions are common concerns about diet and physical activity to do with cancer.

WHAT ARE ANTIOXIDANTS[2], AND WHAT DO THEY HAVE TO DO WITH CANCER ?

The body seems to use certain nutrients in vegetables and fruits to protect against damage to tissues[3] that happens constantly as a result of normal metabolism[4] (oxidation). Because such damage is linked with increased cancer risk, the so-called antioxidant nutrients are thought to protect against cancer. Antioxidants include vitamin C, vitamin E, carotenoids, and many other phytochemicals[5] (chemicals from plants). Clinical studies of antioxidant supplements are currently under way but have not yet proven to reduce cancer risk from vitamin or mineral supplements. To reduce cancer risk, the best advice at present is to get your antioxidants through food sources, rather than supplements.

■ note ■

1) contradictory or conflicting results：矛盾した結論．

2) antioxidant [ǽntiɑ́ksidnt]：抗酸化物質（活性酸素とフリーラジカルによる体内の酸化ストレスを抑制する物質）．

3) tissues：組織（ex. connective [muscular, nervous] tissue 結合［筋肉, 神経］組織）．

4) metabolism：代謝．

5) phytochemicals：植物由来の栄養素．

WILL EATING LESS FAT LOWER CANCER RISK ?

There is little evidence that the total amount of fat a person eats affects cancer risk. But diets high in fat tend to be high in calories and may contribute to obesity, which in turn is linked with an increased risk of several types of cancer. There is evidence that certain types of fats, such as saturated fats[1], may increase cancer risk. There is little evidence, however, that other types of fat (omega-3 fatty acids[2], found mainly in fish), monounsaturated fatty acids[3] (found in olive and canola oils), or polyunsaturated fats[4] reduce cancer risk.

WHAT IS DIETARY FIBER, AND CAN IT PREVENT CANCER ?

Dietary fiber include a wide variety of plant carbohydrates that humans cannot digest. Specific categories of fiber are "soluble" (like oat bran) or "insoluble" (like wheat bran and cellulose). Soluble fiber helps to reduce blood cholesterol, which lower the risk of coronary heart disease[5]. Links between fiber and cancer risk are weak, but eating these foods is still recom-

---

■ note ■

1) saturated fats：飽和脂肪（分子中に炭素の二重結合をもたない脂肪. 獣肉や乳製品に多い）.

2) omega-3 fatty acids：多価不飽和脂肪酸の一種. 背の青い魚 (fish with colored flesh, like salmon, sardines or others) に豊富に含まれる.

3) monounsaturated fatty acids：単価不飽和脂肪酸.

4) polyunsaturated fats：多価不飽和脂肪.

5) coronary heart disease：冠状動脈疾患による心臓病.

mended.

DOES EATING FISH PROTECT AGAINST CANCER ?

Fish is a rich source of omega-3 fatty acids. Studies in animals have found that these fatty acids suppress cancer information or slow down cancer growth, but there is limited evidence of a possible benefit in humans.

CAN GARLIC PREVENT CANCER ?

The health benefits of the allium[1] compounds contained in garlic and other vegetables in the onion family have been publicized widely. Garlic is currently under study for its ability to reduce cancer risk. There is not enough at this time to support a specific role for this vegetable in cancer prevention.

IF OUR GENES[2] DETERMINE CANCER RISK, HOW CAN DIET HELP PREVENT CANCER ?

Damage to the genes that control cell growth can be either inherited or acquired during life. Certain types of mutations[3] or genetic damage can increase the risk of cancer. Nutrients in the

■ note ■

1) allium：アリウム属（ネギ属）．

2) genes [dʒíːnz]：遺伝子（cf. genetic damage 遺伝子の損傷）．

3) mutation：突然変異．

note

1) cruciferous vegetables：アブラナ（十字花）科の野菜.

2) Brussels sprout：芽キャベツ.

3) colorectal cancer：結腸, 直腸のがん.

4) bladder cancer：膀胱がん.

5) dilute：薄める.

6) urine [júərən]：尿.

diet can protect DNA from being damaged.

The interaction between diet and genetic factors is an important and complex topic, and a great deal of research is under way in this area.

WHAT ARE CRUCIFEROUS VEGETABLES[1]?

Cruciferous vegetables belong to the cabbage family and include broccoli, cauliflower, and Brussels sprouts[2]. These vegetables contain compounds thought to reduce the risk for colorectal cancer[3]. The best evidence suggests that eating a wide variety of vegetables, including cruciferous and other vegetables, reduces cancer risk.

HOW MUCH WATER AND OTHER FLUIDS SHOULD I DRINK ?

Drinking water and other liquids may reduce the risk of bladder cancer[4], as water dilutes[5] the concentration of cancer-causing agents in the urine[6] and shortens the time in which they are in contact with the bladder lining. Drinking at least 8 cups of liquid a day is usually recommended, and some studies show that even more may be helpful.

References
- McGinnis JM, Foege WH. Actual causes of death in the United States. *JAMA*. 1993 ; 270 : 2207-2212.
- Bergstrom A, Pisani P, Tenet V, et al. Overweight as an avoidable cause of cancer in Europe. *Int J Cancer*. 2001 ; 91 : 421-430.
- Vainio H, Bianchini F. *Weight Control and Physical Activity*, vol. 6. Lyon, France : International Agency for Research Cancer Press ; 2002.
- Czene K, Lichtenstein P, Hemminki K. Environmental and heritable causes of cancer among 9.6 million individuals in the Swedish Family-Cancer Database. *Int J Cancer*, 2002 ; 99 : 260-266.
- World Cancer Research Fund and American Institute for Cancer Research. Food, Nutrition and the Prevention of Cancer : A Global Perspective. Washington, DC : World Cancer Research Fund and American Institute for Cancer Research ; 1997.
- Friedenreich CM. Physical activity and cancer prevention : from observational to intervention research. *ii* 2001 ; 10 : 287-301.

◆ EXERCISES ◆

(1) Match the words.

1) reduce   2) whole grain   3) poultry
4) beverage   5) evidence   6) tissue
7) recommend   8) maintain

a) a hot or cold drink
b) the material forming animal or plant cells
c) birds such as chickens and ducks kept on farms
d) facts that make you believe that something is true
e) make a level or rate stay the same
f) decrease, or make smaller or less in amount
g) the corn, wheat or rice that are not refined
h) advise someone to do something

(2) Answer the questions.
  1) Give 3 points to maintain a healthy weight.
  2) Explain what vigorous physical activities are, and give at least 3 examples.
  3) To reduce calorie intake and cancer-causing agents, what kind of preparation is preferable for preparing meats ?
  4) Why is the recommended limit of alcohol different between men and women ? Explain.
  5) Does the author recommend antioxidant supplements rather than food sources ? Answer by yes or no, and tell the reason.

◆ ANSWERS ◆

(1)
1) f 2) g 3) c 4) a 5) d 6) b 7) h 8) e

(2)
1) Balance calorie intake with physical activity, avoid excessive weight gain, and keep a healthy weight throughout life.
2) Vigorous activities generally use large muscle groups and cause faster heart rate, deeper and faster breathing, and sweating. The examples are jogging, running, aerobic dance, soccer, lacrosse, or swimming.
3) Baking, poaching, steaming, or stewing. They produce less calories rather than frying or grilling.
4) That is because women are generally smaller in body size and slower in breakdown alcohol.
5) No, because the author says that clinical studies of antioxidant supplements have not yet proven to reduce cancer risk.

3 DO YOU HAVE PREHYPERTENSION[1]?

■ note ■

1) prehypertension：前高血圧症.
2) The National High Blood Pressure Education Program：米国高血圧症対策指導計画.
3) stricter rules：従来よりも厳格な規定.
4) public awareness：社会の関心.
5) hypertension：高血圧症.
6) diagnose：診断する.
7) reading：記録.
8) mmHg：millimeter(s) of mercury；(血圧計の) 水銀柱の目盛＝血圧の数値.
9) level：数値, 測定値.
10) systolic pressure：心臓収縮期の血圧（最高血圧）.
11) contract：収縮する ↔ relax：弛緩する.
12) diastolic pressure：心臓拡張期の血圧（最低血圧）.
13) above ↔ below cf. upper ↔ lower

In 2003, new blood pressure guidelines gave us a wake up call. The National High Blood Pressure Education Program[2] released stricter rules[3].

Their goal was to increase public awareness[4] of hypertension[5] prevention and treatment. A new blood pressure section called prehypertension was added.

Blood pressure levels that had been called normal now became prehypertensive.

New Blood Pressure Standards Hypertension, or high blood pressure, is diagnosed[6] when a blood pressure reading[7] of 140/90 mmHg[8] or greater is noted. The level[9] must be seen on at least two readings to be officially diagnosed. The upper number is the systolic pressure[10] when your heart contracts[11]. The lower number is the diastolic pressure[12] when your heart relaxes.

If your blood pressure was 139/89 mmHg or below[13], it was considered normal.

With 2003 guidelines, only a reading below 120/80 mmHg is considered normal. When your blood pressure is slightly higher than this, you have prehypertension.

Prehypertension Risk

Prehypertensive patients are more likely to develop full-blown[1] hypertension. They are also more likely to develop associated health problems[2]. Heart disease, stroke, kidney disease, blindness, and Alzheimer's disease[3] are all associated with hypertension.

Studies indicate cardiovascular risk increases as blood pressure rises above 115/75 mmHg. In fact, your risk doubles with every 20 mmHg rise[4] in systolic pressure[5] or with every 10 mmHg rise in diastolic pressure.

Who Should Get Screened ?

According to the National High Blood Pressure Education Program, everyone should have a blood pressure check at least once every two years[6]. If your blood pressure is above normal (that is, higher than 120/80 mmHg), your doctor may recommend that you have it rechecked more often. People at increased risk for hyper-

■ note ■

1) full-blown：本格的な，末期の．
2) associated health problems：合併症の症状．
3) Alzheimer's disease：アルツハイマー病．

4) rise：上昇 ↔ drop：下降．
5) with every 20 mmHg rise in systolic pressure：最高血圧が 20 上昇するごとに．

6) once every two years：1 年おきに．

tension may also need more frequent[1] readings. Risk factors include a family history of the condition[2], African American race, above-normal weight, or age greater than 50.

Prehypertension Treatment

Unlike hypertension, prehypertension treatment does not usually include drugs. The mainstay[3] of therapy for prehypertension is lifestyle changes[4]. The following changes can help to slow or prevent progression to hypertension. The National High Blood Pressure Education Program recommends:

LOSE EXCESS WEIGHT.

Studies show that each 10 pounds of weight loss is associated with an average drop in systolic blood pressure of up to about 10 millimeters of mercury.

INCREASE PHYSICAL ACTIVITY TO AT LEAST 30 MINUTES MOST DAYS OF THE WEEK.

First get your doctor's approval if you're not accustomed to exercise[5].

■ note ■

1) frequent：頻繁な．

2) family history of the condition：家族の病歴．

3) mainstay：かなめ，中心．

4) lifestyle changes：生活習慣の改善．

5) be not accustomed to exercise：体を動かす習慣がない．

EAT A HEALTHFUL DIET.

　Daily food intake should be low in[1] saturated fat and cholesterol, and rich in whole grains, fruits and vegetables, and low fat dairy foods.

　Reduce salt intake to no more than 2.4 grams (g) of sodium[2] (the equivalent[3] of about a teaspoon of table salt) a day.

　Limit alcohol use. This means no more than two drinks a day for men or one for women.

　The National High Blood Pressure Education Program released the new guidelines to emphasize the need for more aggressive[4] prevention, detection[5], and treatment. Presently, over 50 million people in America have high blood pressure and an estimated 45 million more have prehypertension. If we don't take action[6] now, 90% of us will likely develop high blood pressure during our lives. In order to be free from[7] fearful epidemic[8] of hypertension, prevention is urgently needed.

(Modified from Chobanian AV, Bakris GL, Black HR, et al. The seventh report of the Joint National Committee on prevention, detection, evaluation, and treatment of high blood pressure. *JAMA*. 2003 ; 289 : 2560-2572.)

■ note ■

1) be low in〜 : 〜が少ない
　↔be rich in〜 : 〜が豊富である.

2) sodium : ナトリウム. (Na)

3) the equivalent : 同量, 等価値.

4) aggressive : 積極的な.

5) detection : 発見, 検出.

6) take action : 措置をとる.

7) be free from〜 : 〜の心配がなくなる.

8) epidemic : 多発, 蔓延. (まんえん)

◆ EXERCISES ◆

1) What is the new blood pressure section called ? (   )
2) Blood pressure readings :

    (   ) systolic / (   ) diastolic   ⟶   diagnosis
    below (   ) / (   ) mmHg   ⟶   (   )
    above 120   / 80 mmHg, even slightly   ⟶   (   )

3) Everyone should have a blood pressure (   ) more than once every (   ) years.
4) In case of prehypertension treatment, doctors usually recommend (   ) changes, instead of drugs. They will advise you to lose excess (   ), increase (   ) activity, and to eat a healthful (   ).
5) Daily food intake should be (   ) in saturated (   ) and cholesterol, but (   ) in whole grains, (   ) and vegetables, and low fat (   ) foods.

◆ ANSWERS ◆

1) prehypertension
2) upper/lower/120/80/normal/prehypertensive
3) check/two
4) lifestyle/weight/physical/diet
5) low/fat/rich/fruits/dairy

4 FOLATE, A NUTRIENT FOR ALL AGES

What is folate ?

Folate is a water-soluble B-complex vitamin that occurs naturally in food.

A key observation of researcher Lucy Wills, nearly 70 years ago, led to the identification[1] of folate as the nutrient needed to prevent anemia[2] in pregnancy[3]. Dr. Wills demonstrated that this type of anemia could be corrected[4] with a yeast extract[5]. Folate was identified[6] as the corrective substance[7] in yeast extract in the late 1930s, and was also extracted from spinach leaves in 1941.

Folate in the diet may reduce the risk of several serious diseases

Folate helps produce and maintain new cells. Folate is needed to make DNA[8] and RNA[9], the building blocks of cells.

Early research suggests that getting plenty of folate in the diet may reduce the risk of several serious diseases. It may help prevent heart diseases and stroke by interfering with substances that clog[10] the arteries[11]. Lack of folate affects

■ note ■

1) identification：認定
2) anemia：貧血症
3) pregnancy：妊娠期間
4) correct：治療する，治す
5) yeast extract：酵母エキス
6) identify：確認する
7) corrective substance：調整物質

8) DNA：デオキシリボ核酸
9) RNA：リボ核酸

10) clog：詰まらせる，塞ぐ
11) artery：動脈

■ n o t e ■

1) colon：結腸

2) bearing children：出産

3) spine：脊髄，背骨

4) citrus：柑橘類

5) synthetic form：合成体

6) fortified food：強化食品

the growth of red blood cells. This can lead to anemia, a condition in which the blood can't carry enough oxygen. Anemia can make you feel tired and have a lack of energy.

Folate also helps prevent changes to DNA that may lead to cancer of colon$_{1)}$ by helping to protect cells in the colon.

Women capable of bearing children$_{2)}$ need plenty of folate

Folate is most important in the first weeks of pregnancy. This is when an unborn baby's spine$_{3)}$ and brain are developing. During this time, the women may not know she is pregnant, and the unborn baby needs folate to develop properly.

What foods provide folate ?

Folate gets its name from the Latin word "folium" for leaf. Leafy green vegetables (like spinach and turnip greens), fruits (like citrus$_{4)}$ fruits and juices), and dried beans and peas are all natural sources of folate.

Folic acid is the synthetic form$_{5)}$ of folate that is found in supplements and is added to fortified foods$_{6)}$. In USA, the Food and Drug Administra-

48

tion (FDA)1) published regulations in 1996, requiring the addition of folic acid to enriched2) breads, cereals, flours, corn meals, pastas, rice, and other grain products. Since cereals and grains are widely consumed in the U.S., these products have become a very important contributor3) of folic acid in the American diet.

How much folate do you need ?

　　Our body cannot make folate. It has to get it from food. Foods in the bread, cereal, rice and pasta group contain folate, so they are now all fortified with folate in USA. A variety of fruits and vegetables are good for your diet and eating them makes getting enough folate easier than you think.

　　However, too much of a good thing can be harmful. Folate in doses above 1,000 micrograms can conceal a deficiency4) of vitamin B_{12}. This deficiency can cause permanent nerve damage and paralysis5).

　　That is why good nutrition is so important. Although folate is definitely necessary for our body, it is not the one and only kind of nutrient we need to include in our daily food intake. The

---

■ n o t e ■

1) Food and Drug Administration (FDA)：食・医薬品局（米）

2) enriched：強化された

3) become a contributor：〜に一役買っている

4) deficiency：欠乏症

5) paralysis：麻痺

■ note ■

1) requirement：必要量

following tables will show you the difference of the amount of folate required for different physical conditions. Find your folate requirement₁₎, and try to take a variety of food at every meal ; this will help you to get all the vitamins, minerals and fiber your body needs every day.

TABLE 1   RDA* FOR FOLATE FOR CHILDREN AND ADULTS

Age (years)	Males and Females (μg/day)	Pregnancy (μg/day)	Lactation (μg/day)
1〜3	150	N/A	N/A
4〜8	200	N/A	N/A
9〜13	300	N/A	N/A
14〜18	400	600	500
19+	400	600	500

＊：Recommended Dietary Allowances；推奨量

TABLE 2   AI** FOR FOLATE FOR INFANTS

Age (months)	Males and Females (μg/day)
0 to 6	65
7 to 12	80

＊＊：Adequate Intake；目安量

Why women of childbearing age and pregnant women have a special need for folate ?

As folic acid is especially needed during periods of rapid cell division and growth, adequate folate intake during the periconceptual period[1], the time just before and after a woman becomes pregnant, protects against neural tube defects[2]. Neural tube defects result in malformations[3] of the spine (spina bifida[4]), skull[5], and brain (anencephaly[6]).

Since January 1998, when the folate food fortification program took effect, data suggest that there has been a significant[7] reduction in neural tube birth defects[8]. Women who could become pregnant are advised to eat foods fortified with folic acid or take a folic acid supplement in addition to eating folate-rich foods to reduce the risk of these serious birth defects.

Folic acid and cancer

Folate is involved in the synthesis, repair, and function of DNA, our genetic map, and there is some evidence that a deficiency of folate can cause damage to DNA that may lead to cancer.

■ n o t e ■

1) periconceptual period：受胎前後の期間
2) neural tube defect：神経管欠損症
3) malformation：奇形
4) spina bifida：二分脊椎症，脊椎分裂
5) skull：頭骨，頭蓋骨
6) anencephaly：無脳症，無頭蓋症
7) significant：(医) 著しい
8) birth defect：先天性欠損 (症)

■ note ■

1) breast (cancer)：乳（腺）（がん）

2) pancreatic (cancer)：膵臓（がん）

Several studies have associated diets low in folate with increased risk of breast[1], pancreatic[2], and colon cancer. Over 88,000 women enrolled in the Nurses' Health Study who were free of cancer in 1980 were followed from 1980 through 1994. Researchers found that women ages 55 to 69 years in this study who took multivitamins containing folic acid for more than 15 years had a markedly lower risk of developing colon cancer. Findings from over 14,000 subjects followed for 20 years suggest that men who do not consume alcohol and whose diets provide the recommended intake of folate are less likely to develop colon cancer. However, associations between diet and disease do not indicate a direct cause.

Researchers are continuing to investigate whether enhanced folate intake from foods or folic acid supplements may reduce the risk of cancer. Until results from such clinical trials are available, folic acid supplements should not be recommended to reduce the risk of cancer.

Caution about folic acid supplements

Intake of supplemental folic acid should not exceed 1,000 micrograms (μg) per day to prevent folic acid from triggering[1] symptoms of vitamin B₁₂ deficiency. Folic acid supplements can correct the anemia associated with vitamin B₁₂ deficiency. Unfortunately, however, folic acid will not correct changes in the nervous system that result from vitamin B₁₂ deficiency. Permanent nerve damage can occur if vitamin B₁₂ deficiency is not treated.

The Institute of Medicine has established a tolerable upper intake level (UL)[2] for folate from fortified foods or supplements (i.e. folic acid) for ages one and above. Intakes above this level increase the risk of adverse health effects. In adults, supplemental folic acid should not exceed the UL to prevent folic acid from triggering symptoms of vitamin B₁₂ deficiency. It is important to recognize that the UL refers to the amount of synthetic folate (i.e. folic acid) being consumed per day from fortified foods and/or supplements.

■ note ■

1) trigger：誘発する

2) tolerable upper intake：摂取許容量の上限

■ note ■

Selecting a healthful diet

As the 2000 Dietary Guidelines for Americans states, "Different foods contain different nutrients and other healthful substances. No single food can supply all the nutrients in the amounts you need". Green leafy vegetables, dried beans and peas, and many other types of vegetables and fruits provide folate.

There is no health risk, and no UL, for natural sources of folate found in food. Before thinking about taking a folic acid supplement, it is important to try to include adequate sources of dietary folate and fortified food sources of folic acid in your daily meals.

■ **Lucy Wills** ■

イギリスの科学者 (1888-1964)．1911 年 Cambridge 大学卒業（植物学専攻）．実務を経て 1920 年には London School of Medicine for Women を卒業．1920 年代後半より医師としてインドで妊娠時の貧血の調査・研究を続け，1937 年に酵母菌から有効成分を発見し，ビタミン M と命名．1941 年にホウレンソウの葉から発見された乳酸菌の増殖因子の成分が，これと同一であると証明され，folic acid（葉酸）とよばれるようになった．

◆ EXERCISES ◆

1) Folate is a (　　) –soluble (　　) vitamin, and was first identified as the (　　) needed to prevent (　　) in pregnancy.
Folate helps produce and maintain new cells; it is needed to make DNA and RNA, the building blocks of cells.

2) Our body cannot make folate. We must get it from (　　).
Folic acid is the synthetic form of folate, that is found in supplements and added to (　　) foods.
In order to avoid the risk of B_{12} deficiency, the intake of supplemental folic acid should not exceed (　　). Try to include (　　) and fortified food sources of (　　), before thinking about taking a folic acid (　　).

◆ ANSWERS ◆

1) water/B/nutrient/anemia

2) food/fortified/UL/folate/folic acid/supplements

★ Please encourage a young woman to take lots of natural sources of folate. She is 24, married and may not know she is pregnant yet.

   a. What should she eat ?
   b. How much folate should she take every day ?
   c. Can you tell her why it is very important for her to take folate now ?

★ a. Read "What foods provide folate ?", and the last paragraph once again !
   b. Look up at Table 1, on page 50.
   c. See the 3rd and the 6th paragraghs.

Chapter 4

DIETITAN'S MESSAGE

In the field of nutrition, one thing that is always constant is change. Nutrition research and development of treatment for health issues, food production and distribution, equipment, food safety will continue to evolve and improve our lives. Controversy will always be a part of nutrition recommendations and moderation may become the truth for everyone with good nutrition practices. However, the field of nutrition is always fascinating and of interest to people around the world. I genuinely hope you enjoy this field of study and find this chapter useful in your practice and lives.

1 ADULT LEARNING

Adult learning in a well-run dietary department includes continuing education for all staff members.
Adults learn through a combination of learning styles including visual, auditory or kinesthetic (learning by doing).

Learners are likely to refine[1]:
　…10% of what they read
　…20% of what they hear
　…30% of what they see
　…50% of what they see and hear
　…70% of what they discuss
　…80% of what they experience personally, and
　…95% of what they teach to someone else.

The more the learner participates and gets involved, the higher the likelihood the information will be retained[2]. Include participation and discussion as well as auditory, visual, and kinesthetic learning (practice/doing) in each training experience for maximum retention. Final tip, KEEP IT SIMPLE, so everyone understands.

Suggested inservice[3] topics

① emergency meal plan and menus

② portion control

③ proper lifting[4]

④ fire/disaster plans

⑤ patient's rights

⑥ infection control

⑦ documentation

⑧ menus and special diet concerns

⑨ FIFO (first in, first out)

⑩ cleaning instructions

⑪ food preparation and handling

⑫ meal service and dining

⑬ sanitation and safety

Documentation in medical charts frequently is done with this abbreviation.

S…Subjective from client

O…Objective information

A…Assessment

P…Plan

DIETITIAN'S MESSAGE

A more current form of documentation includes nutrition diagnosis[5]. This is a PES evaluation for clients in the nutrition care process.

　P...Problem
　E...Etiology[6]
　S...Signs and Symptoms

A rote[7] with standardized language including terminology[8], intervention[9], monitoring, and evaluation to benefit clients.

■ n o t e ■

1) refine : to improve (by gradually making slight changes to it)
2) retain (v) : to keep something or continue to have something
　 (cf : (n) retention)
3) inservice : training at work on the job
4) proper lifting : how to lift heavy items so one doesn't get hurt
5) diagnosis : the process or result of finding out what illness a person has
6) etiology : the cause of a disease
7) rote : repeating something many times
8) terminology : the technical words or expressions
9) intervention : the act of doing something to try (and stop) an argument or dealing with a problem

2 TIPS FOR DIETITIANS

As a dietitian, remember there are different approaches with patients and use what works for you and each individual patient or their significant others (family). Watch other professionals to get ideas to improve your skills including peer review[1], group presentations and grand rounds with other medical staff. National and international conferences can be another way to improve your skills as a dietitian and speaker.

Sometimes the best ideas in food service come from your employees so be sure to listen to their suggestions.

Prioritize[2] your day so you can accomplish your goals.

Volunteer at least once a year for a good cause. It is a wonderful way to meet others and to broaden your experiences with civic organizations. If you are not comfortable speaking with groups or individuals, join a group such as Toastmasters to improve your skills.

Look for the good in others. Take care of your staff and don't be unreasonable with your requests. Be fair to your staff and honest in business practices.

Make friends with others. Find a hobby you enjoy. Practice what you preach and be a good example for others such as be on time to work. Encourage others. Give praise when it is deserved.

Visit other hospitals or schools for ideas and start a journal club to meet other dietitians and medical staff and this will help you keep current with continuing education.

Take an interest in your clients and their culture and foods. Try a new recipe if you can find something different. Take a trip to learn about other cultures and foods.

Stick to deadlines as much as possible. Delegate$_{3)}$ whenever you can. Lead and try to be first (best) in everything you do.

Your reputation follows and precedes you so do the right thing always. Do your job right the first time and ahead of the deadline so you can review your work and make corrections if necessary.

Be an expert. Admit if you don't know but go find out so you become the expert.

If an opportunity to gain skills in computers, management, purchasing, supervision is available, please take the opportunity even if you have to volunteer. Ask questions and continue your education as

DIETITIAN'S MESSAGE

you can never know it all but remember to share your expertise[4] with others. Try new things such as telemedicine[5], conference calls[6] for education, and other new technology applications in nutrition.

5

Live everyday like it's your last. Relax as any situation could be worse. Ask yourself if it will matter in a week, a year, or 5 years. If not, then inhale and exhale and don't worry.

■ n o t e ■

1) peer review：査読，論文発表前の，他の研究者による内容の吟味や調査．
2) prioritize：優先順位をつける．
3) delegate：率先する．
4) expertise：専門的知識，学術調査報告．
5) telemedicine：遠隔医療．
6) conference calls：（3人以上の）電話会議．

3   YOU CAN FIND IT

With the Internet you can find accurate and inaccurate nutrition information. Here are some recommended sites for good information, useful to you, regardless of your citizenship. Cyberspace knows no borders or boundaries.

http://www.eatright.org　　　　　（American Dietetic Association）
http://www.pueblo.gsa.gov
　　　　　（Consumer information children, health, food and nutrition）
http://www.cihi.ca　　　（Canadian Institute for Health Information）
http://www.cdc.gov　（Centers for Disease Control and Prevention）
http://www.nal.usda.gov/fnic/
　　　　　　　　　　　（Food and Nutrition Information Center）
http://www.nih.gov　　　　　　　（National Institutes of Health）
http://www.feinberg.northwestern.edu/nutrition/fact-sheets.html
　　　　　　　　　　　　　　　　　　　（Northwestern University）
http://ods.od.nih.gov/Health_Information/Vitamin_and_Mineral_
　Supplement_Fact_Sheets.aspx.
　　（National Institutes of Health, Office of Dietary Supplements）
http://www.ausport.gov.au/ais/nutrition/factsheets
　　　　　　　　　　　　　　　　（Australian Institute of Sports）
http://www.glutenfree.com/newsletter　　　　（glutenfree. com）

APPENDIX

FIGURE
    1   OUR DIGESTIVE SYSTEM
    2   BRAIN AND HEART

TABLE
    1   ESSENTIAL NUTRIENTS FOR GOOD HEALTH

FIGURE 1 OUR DIGESTIVE SYSTEM

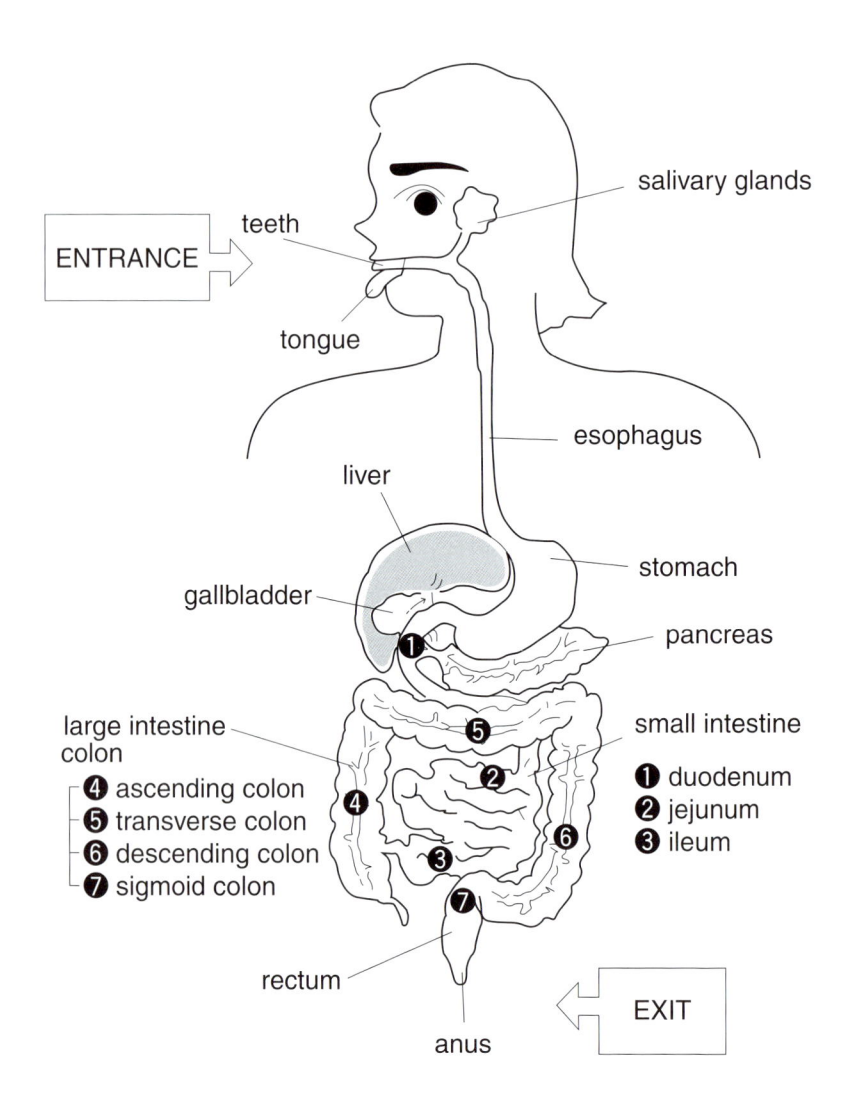

APPENDIX

FIGURE 2 BRAIN AND HEART

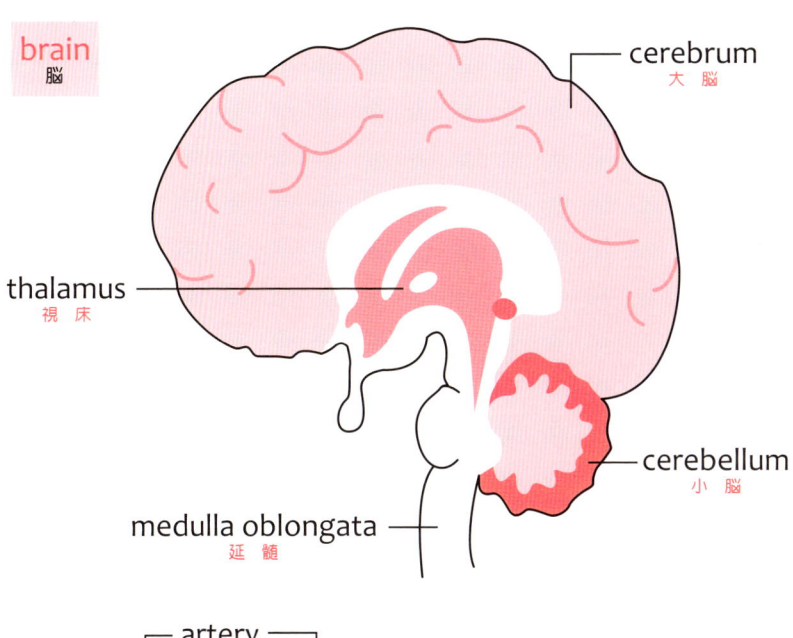

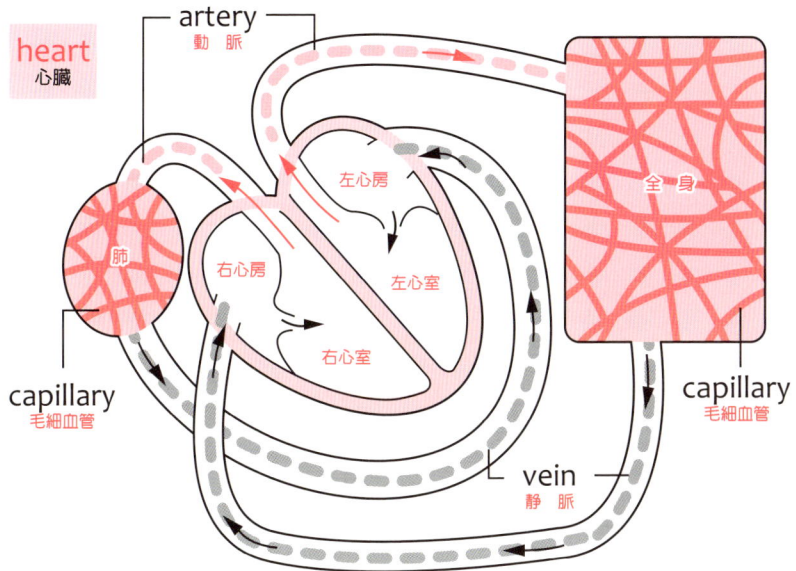

brain
脳

cerebrum
大脳

thalamus
視床

cerebellum
小脳

medulla oblongata
延髄

heart
心臓

artery
動脈

左心房
右心房
左心室
右心室
肺
全身

capillary
毛細血管

capillary
毛細血管

vein
静脈

67

APPENDIX

TABLE 1 ESSENTIAL NUTRIENTS FOR GOOD HEALTH

Nutrient : Why It's Needed	Major Dietary Sources
PROTEIN : Required for growth maintenance and repair of body tissues.	Meat, poultry, fish, eggs, milk and milk products, soybeans, beans, peas, grains and nuts. (g)
CARBOHYDRATE : Supplies energy for physical activity, bodily processes, and warmth.	Starches ; Cereals and cereal products, such as bread, spaghetti, macaroni, noodles and baked goods. Sugars ; sugar, syrops, jam, honey, candy, confections and other sweets. (g)
LIPIDS : Provides an average energy intake of 9 kcal/gram which is twice that of carbohydrate or protein at 4 kcal/gram. A minimum amount of dietary fat is necessary to facilitate absorption of fat-soluble vitamins (A, D, E and K) and carotenoids, and is also necessary to provide insulation that prevents heat loss and protects vital organs from shock due to ordinary activities.	
Fatty Acid (1) **Saturated** ; has maximum number of hydrogens on the carbon chain solid at room temperature, high melting point	Meats, poultry, and dairy foods ; coconuts and palm oils.
(2) **Trans** ; product of hydrogenation which increases the saturation of fatty acids within oils and converts natural cis to trans configuration ; industrially processed to enhance product taste, stability and shelf life.	Commercially fried or baked foods, margarine, and vegetable shortenings.

68

Nutrient : Why It's Needed	Major Dietary Sources
(3) **Monounsaturated** ; contain one double bond. Liquid at room temperature.	Olive, peanut and canola oils, nuts, avocados, and olives.
(4) **Polyunsaturated** ; contain two or more double bonds. Liquid at room temperature.	Corn, soybean, safflower and sunflower seed oils, and fish.

Omega 3 Fatty Acids
• Linolenic acid
  (18 : 3 omega 3)
• Eicosapentaenoic acid
  (20 : 5 omega 3) (EPA)
• Docosahexaenoic acid
  (22 : 6 omega 3) (DHA)
	Salmon, mackerel, herring, flaxseed, walnuts, walnut oil, soybean and soybean oil.

Omega 6 Fatty Acids
• Linoleic acid
  (18 : 2 omega 6)
• Arachidonic fatty acid
  (20 : 4 omega 6)
	Corn, soybean and safflower margarine and oils.

Essential Fatty Acids (must be obtained from the diet)
• Linoleic acid
  (18 : 2 omega 6)
• Linolenic acid
  (18 : 3 omega 3)	

Tryglycerides	Neutral esters of glycerol and fatty acids most contain different types of fatty acids (mixed) most common form of dietary fats and oils.	
VITAMIN A (Retinol) : Important for normal growth in children. Improves night vision. Essential for healthy skin, eyes and hair.	Liver, deep yellow and dark leafy green vegetables, egg yolk, butter, and fortified margarine. (g)

APPENDIX

Nutrient : Why It's Needed	Major Dietary Sources
VITAMIN B$_1$ (thiamine) : Helps to convert sugar to energy in the muscles and bones. Necessary for proper function of heart and nervous systems.	Lean pork, liver, heart, kidney, dried beans and peas, whole grain, enriched breads and cereals. (mg)
VITAMIN B$_2$ (ribofravin) : Essential for building and maintaining body tissues. Promotes healthy skin and hair. Protects against cancer.	Milk and milk products, liver, dried yeast, enriched breads and cereals. (mg)
VITAMIN B$_6$ (Pyridoxine) : Is a coenzyme for enzymes involved in amino acid metabolism. Vitamin B$_6$ supplements in pharmacologic doses have been used to treat carpal tunnel syndrome, premenstrual syndrome, and depression. : is easily destroyed in processing foods. Fresh meats and raw produce also provide greater levels of vitamin B$_6$ than their processed counterparts.	Liver, oatmeal, banana, salmon, chicken meat, potatoes. (mg)
VITAMIN B$_{12}$ (cobalamin) : Helps body form red blood cells. Improves memory and concentration. Protects against allergens and blood vessels.	Lean meat, liver, kidney salt-water fish, milk and oysters. (μg)
VITAMIN C (Ascorbic Acid) : Is a water-soluble antioxidant responsible for maintaining iron preserving activity of the hundreds of enzymes that contain iron at the catalytic site. Tissues most sensitive to vitamin C status are those which contain large amounts of collagen such as blood vessels and capillaries, bone, and scar tissue. : is sensitive to destruction by exposure to light, heat, air, or pro-oxidant mineral such as iron or copper. To maximize vitamin C content of dietary sources, these foods should be stored in sealed containers under refrigeration and prepared by methods requiring low temperatures and minimal cooking time.	Orange juice, grapefruit juice, papaya, strawberries,···vitamin C is found only in foods of plant origin. Consumption of more than 100 mg vitamin C daily in supplement form may reduce the severity and duration of colds when consumed with onset of symptoms. To maintain serum vitamin C levels in smokers, 100 mg of vitamin C daily is required.

APPENDIX

Nutrient : Why It's Needed	Major Dietary Sources
VITAMIN D : Helps the body utilize calcium and phosphorus. Protects against osteoporosis. Sunlight is necessary for our bodies to synthesize V. D.	Milk, cod liver oil, salmon, tuna and yolk. (μg)
VITAMIN E (Tocopherol) : Plays a key role in preventing cellular injury from oxidative stress associated with premature aging, cataracts, uncontrolled diabetes, cardiovascular disease, inflammation, and infection. : is heat-stable, the high temperatures used in frying can destroy the vitamin. Regular consumption of processed grain products may contribute to a marginal vitamin E intake. Additionally, very low-fat intakes (<15% total energy) also decrease vitamin E.	Wheat germ oil, wheat germ, sunflower seeds, mango, avocado. Vitamin E requirements are measured in milligrams (mg). However, vitamin E content is measured in International Units (IU) on food labels. To convert IU to mg, one IU of vitamin E is equivalent to 67 mg.
PANTOTHENIC ACID : Necessary for the body's use of carbohydrates, fats and protein. Aids in the reduction of stress. Lowers cholesterol levels.	Almost universally present in plant and animal tissue. (mg)
FOLATE (folacin or folic acid) : Helps produce and maintain new cells. : is especially important during periods of rapid cell division and growth such as infancy and pregnancy. : is needed to make DNA and RNA, the building blocks of cells, and it also helps prevent changes to DNA that may lead to cancer. Both adults and children need folate to make normal red blood cells and prevent anemia. : is also essential for the metabolism of homocysteine, and helps maintain normal levels of this amino acid. Risk of folate deficiency is highest among women, elderly adults, smokers, and alcoholics. : is highly sensitive to destruction by heat and light. Methods of cooking, processing or food storage can result in destruction of 50-95% of the folate content of food.	Leafy green vegetables (spinach and turnip greens), liver (chicken, beef), dried beans and peas, fruits (citrus fruits and juices) (μg)

APPENDIX

Nutrient : Why It's Needed	Major Dietary Sources
NIACHIN : Necessary for converting food to energy. Aids the digestion and nervous system.	Tuna, liver, lean meat, fish, poultry and peas. (mg)
BIOTIN : Prevents hair from graying and helps to prevent baldness. Aids in clotting of blood.	Egg yolk, milk, liver and green vegetables. (μg)
CALCIUM (Ca) : Is the most abundant mineral in the human body, and has several important functions. : more than 99% of total body calcium is stored in the bones and teeth where it functions to support their structure. The remaining 1% is found throughout the body in blood, muscle, and the fluid between cells. : is needed for muscle contraction, blood vessel contraction and expansion, the secretion of hormones and enzymes, and sending messages through the nervous system. : bone undergoes continuous remodeling, with breakdown of bone and bone formation. The balance between them changes as people age. During childhood there is a higher amount of bone formation and less breakdown. In aging adults, particularly among postmenopausal women, bone breakdown exceeds its formation, resulting in bone loss, which increases the risk for osteoporosis (a disorder characterized by porous, weak bones). : adequate vitamin D intake from food and sun exposure is essential to bone health, and weight bearing exercise also helps maximize bone strength and bone density.	Yogurt, sardines, Cheddar cheese, milk, tofu, spinach. (mg)

Nutrient : Why It's Needed	Major Dietary Sources
IRON (Fe) : Is involved in energy metabolism as an oxygen carrier in hemoglobin and as a structural component of cytochromes in electron transport. Can be obtained either as heme iron from beef, lamb, pork and poultry or as nonheme iron from vegetables, whole grains, fortified grain products, and supplements. Heme iron is more bioavailable than nonheme iron because it is a soluble complex absorbed intact by endocytosis. Acidic foods such as tomato sauce or orange juice consumed with a nonheme iron food source such as pasta or breakfast cereal will significantly increase the amount of iron asorbed from the meal. High dose supplements of calcium, zinc, manganese, magnesium or copper reduce iron absorption through competition for mucosal uptake. Tannic acid in coffee and tea also adversely affcts iron absorption.	Red meats, organ meats, shellfish (clams, oysters), pumpkin seeds, sunflower seeds, whole grains, nuts, dried beans. (mg)
IODINE (I) : Involves the synthesis of thyroid hormone. About 60% of the total body pool of iodine is stored in the thyroid gland, and the remainder is found in the blood, ovary, and muscle. Thyroid hormone is necessary for regulation of human growth and development.	Seafood (clams, lobster, oyster, sardines and ocean fish), iodized salt. (μg)
MAGNESIUM (Mg) : Involved with normal function of brain and spinal cord. Helps to prevent kidney and gallstones. Useful in treatment of high blood pressure.	Beans and peas, whole wheat flour, green leafy vegetables, nuts and fig. (mg)

APPENDIX

Nutrient : Why It's Needed	Major Dietary Sources
MANGANESE (Mn) : A cofactor for enzymes involved in hydrolysis, phosphorylation, and transamination.	Wheat germ, nuts, seeds, whole grains, oyster, sweet potatoes, tofu, chocolate, brewed tea and dark molasses, fruits and vegetables such as pineapple, grape juice and tomato juice. (mg)
PHOSPHORUS (P) : Necessary for the body's use of fats and carbohydrates. Acts as a cofactor for many enzymes and activates B-complex vitamins.	Milk, cheese, yolk, meat, fish, poultry, beans, nuts and whole grain cereals. (mg)
POTASSIUM (K) : Necessary for the building of muscle and for normal body growth. Essential for the normal electrical activity of the heart. It assists in the regulation of the acid-base balance, and helps in protein synthesis from amino acids and in carbohydrate metabolism. People on dialysis for kidney failure should avoid consuming too many of these potassium-rich foods. These people require specialized diets to avoid excess potassium in the blood.	Vegetables including broccoli, peas, lima beans, tomatoes, potatoes (especially their skins), sweet potatoes, and winter squashes. Fruits including citrus fruits, cantaloupe, bananas, kiwi, prunes, and apricots. Milk and yogurt, as well as nuts. (mg)
ZINC (Zn) : Serves as a cofactor for over 100 enzymes in the body, especially those involved with the metabolism of protein, carbohydrate, fat and alcohol. Essential for maintenance of DNA and RNA, tissue growth and repair, wound healing, taste acuity, prostaglandin production and blood clotting. Is an integral mineral for fetal development and sperm production. Excess intakes of iron or copper can adversely interfere with zinc absorption. Zinc from meat products is four times more bioavailable than that found in feverous grain foods.	Oysters, beef, liver, crab, seafood, poultry, nuts and seeds, whole grains, tofu, legumes and milk. (mg)

Nutrient : Why It's Needed	Major Dietary Sources
COPPER (Cu) : Is a component of enzymes involved in collagen synthesis. About one third of the total body pool of copper is localized in skeletal muscle, another third is found in brain and liver, and the remaining amount of total body copper is found in bone and other tissues. Since copper is excreted primarily in the bile, diseases of the liver and gall bladder may affect copper balance. High dose supplements of zinc, vitamin C, and iron are contributing causes of marginal copper deficiency.	Organ meats, seafood, nuts, seeds, whole grains, legumes, chocolate, cherries, dried fruits, milk, tea, chicken, and potatoes. (μg)
MOLYBDENUM (Mo) : A cofactor of aldehyde oxidases which are involved in purine and pyrimidine detoxification. Xanthine oxidase is responsible for metabolism of uric acid.	Milk, dried beans, peas, nuts and seeds, eggs, liver, tomatoes, carrots, and meats. (μg)
SELENIUM (Se) : A component of glutathione peroxidases for reducing peroxide free radicals. Also has a role in prostaglandin synthesis. Soil selenium content determines the amount of selenium concentrated in plant sources which can vary as much as 200-fold between crops grown in different regions. Processing of grains decreases the selenium content of the grain products.	Brazil nuts, seafood, kidney, liver, meat, poultry, whole grain pasta, sunflower seeds, oatmeal, nuts, eggs and low-fat dairy products. (μg)

Nutrient : Why It's Needed	Major Dietary Sources
CHROMIUM (Cr) : Was first identified as a component of the "glucose-tolerance factor" required for maintenance of normal blood glucose. Has a role in insulin-dependent activities such as protein and lipid metabolism. Chromium supplementation has been found to improve glucose tolerance in elderly adults who have low blood chromium levels. Milled grains or other processed foods have considerably less chromium content than their unprocessed counterparts. Foods cooked with acid-based sauces in stainless steel pans may obtain additional chromium from some types of cookware.	Whole grains, potatoes, oyster, liver, seafood, cheese, chicken, and meat, brewer's yeast. (μg)
DIETARY FIBER : Consists of nondigestible polysaccharides in plant cell walls. Insoluble and soluble fibers are differentiated by viscosity. Viscosity is beneficial for regulation of blood glucose and of appetite, and may also reduce the quantity of bile acids reabsorbed.	Chick peas, kidney beans, soybeans, rice (brown), whole wheat bagel, all-bran, pumpkin.
WATER : Constitutes about 60% of adult body weight, and is a catalyst for a majority of enzymatic reactions including those involved in nutrient digestion, absorption, transport, and metabolism. It is also required for facilitating excretion of metabolic waste by the kidneys.	

THE SOURCES

■Chapter 1
- http://www.womansday.com

■Chapter 2
- FIVE KEYS to SAFER FOOD MANUAL : WHO
- http://www.extention.iastate.edu/foodsafety/lesson/
- http://www.foodsafety.gov/

■Chapter 3
- http://www.fda.gov/food/guidanceregulation/guidancedocuments
    regulatoryinformation/labelingnutrition/ucm385663.htm#images
- Family Circle, MARCH 2009
- http://www.goodhousekeeping.com/health/
- http://www.cancer.org/
- http://ods.od.nih.gov/Health_Information/Vitamin_and_Mineral_
    Supplement_Fact_Sheets.aspx

■Appendix
- A Step-By-Step Guide : Karen Sullivan, Element Book Inc., Boston
- Northwestern University Medical School NAA Web Site Macronutrients
- http://www.nih.gov/
- http://ods.od.nih.gov/Health_Information/Vitamin_and_Mineral_
    Supplement_Fact_Sheets.aspx

小川 成子
津田塾大学卒業
東京栄養食糧専門学校専任講師，女子栄養大学非常勤講師兼任
翻訳：特許庁委嘱により，英国および米国独占禁止法ほか
共編注：飯野 亮一，学建書院
Best English for Dietitians

山本 厚子
カナダ British Columbia 州立大学大学院修士課程修了
'80 年より香川栄養専門学校栄養士科・女子栄養大学非常勤講師
'85 年同校・同学助教授，'09 年 3 月退職．
共訳：餌取 章男，悪食のサル（Lyall Watson 著），河出書房新社，ほか
共編注：沼田 昌子，北星堂
Food and You

Laura Nihan, Ph. D., R.D.
アメリカ合衆国空軍生物医科学学隊に所属し，'86 年顕彰．
'95 年小児のビタミン A 摂取に関する研究で，Utah 州立大学栄養学部大学院にて Ph.D. 取得．以来，地域の栄養指導プログラムの責任者，また大学および大学院の栄養士養成課程の教員として，アメリカ各地で活躍．
元アメリカ合衆国空軍中佐．初版当時，横須賀海軍病院栄養指導部長．現在ヴァージニア州にて米国退役軍人医療センター栄養指導主任の傍ら，管理栄養士としてカタール国ドーハにて医学研究・栄養指導に従事．米国在外栄養士学会カタール支部代表．
著書：Healthy Heart Shopping Guide, Nutrient-Drug Interactions ほか
American Dietetic Association, American Society for Parenteral and Enteral Nutrition, American Overseas Dietetic Association 会員．

PRACTICAL ENGLISH FOR DIETITIANS　REVISED EDITION

2000 年 2 月 1 日　第 1 版第 1 刷 発行	著　者	小　川　成　子
2003 年 3 月 30 日　第 2 版第 1 刷 発行		山　本　厚　子
2010 年 5 月 31 日　第 3 版第 1 刷 発行		LAURA NIHAN
2013 年 2 月 1 日　第 3 版第 2 刷 発行		
2016 年 2 月 1 日　第 3 版第 3 刷 発行	発行者	木　村　勝　子

発行所　株式会社 学建書院
〒113-0033　東京都文京区本郷 2-13-13　本郷七番館 1F
TEL (03)3816-3888
FAX (03)3814-6679
http://www.gakkenshoin.co.jp
印刷・製本　三報社印刷(株)

ⒸShigeko Ogawa, Atsuko Yamamoto, 2000. Printed in Japan ［検印廃止］

JCOPY 〈(社)出版者著作権管理機構 委託出版物〉
本書の無断複写は著作権法上での例外を除き禁じられています．複写される場合は，そのつど事前に，(社)出版者著作権管理機構（電話 03-3513-6969，FAX 03-3513-6979）の許諾を得てください．

ISBN978-4-7624-2851-7